Eat Yourself Slim

Eat Yourself Slim

Shirley Bright Boody

GRAMERCY PUBLISHING COMPANY • NEW YORK

Dedicated to the many
who have lost so much.

This edition published by Gramercy Publishing Company
a division of Crown Publishers, Inc.
by arrangement with A. S. Barnes and Co., Inc.
c d e f g h

Printed in the United States of America

Contents

Introduction

Nobody wants to be fat and yet there are fifty million fat Americans.

Weight reduction has become a subject of as much public interest as the space program. The methods and procedures are countless and the contradictions are as numerous. They have to be unsuccessful because the number of overweight people is increasing at a greater rate than the total population.

My weight reducing program is sensible and logical. It is a completely new concept based on sound nutrition and healthy eating habits.

The program provides four basic benefits:

(1) Pounds and inches are removed only from the areas where fat has accumulated.

(2) Your weight loss will be permanent.

(3) You need never feel hungry as it includes six eating periods each day, three substantial meals and three snacks.

(4) It will result in a healthier, more youthful body.

The mere mention of dieting conjures up visions of extreme privation, special dietary foods and unappetizir menus. The meals and snacks included in this diet are as accessible as your grocer's shelves and as palatable as last Sunday's dinner.

The program is applicable to men, women and children. It is designed to remove fat deposits only, thus all well-proportioned areas of your body will be unaffected.

I am not an M.D., psychiatrist or psychologist. The references to medical and mental disorders associated with obesity are either common knowledge or information accumulated through my years of observations and collaboration with the medical profession.

I am a dietitian. A dietitian is, "one who is professionally qualified to apply the principles of nutrition to a program of feeding."

Perhaps the most gratifying rewards received from my program relate to health and vitality. It has been my experience that most people will begin to feel better even before they show an appreciable weight loss.

Read this book, practice its theories, and enjoy the rewards of a healthy slender body. You will look younger, feel younger; and you may add years to your life.

1

On Again, Off Again, On Again

The vast number of people who are overweight and have been for ten or more years have exercised their will in a number of adventures in weight reduction. This on again, off again, on again, routine results in discouragement, disillusionment, and frustration, conditioning the obese to accept their "fate." "I was born to be fat." "No diet works for me." "No more, I've tried them all."

A familiar pattern in the life of the heavyweight is periodic qualms of conscience characterized by remorse and self-denial, followed by defiance and indulgence. The cycle repeats itself monotonously until the individual either arrives at the age (generally about sixty) when the flattery of a lithesome shape holds no reward and the years of battling the pounds have exhausted the patience; or the incentives of health, comfort and pride somehow have lost significance.

For each diet or weight loss program you have embraced

you have found reasons for discontinuing or excuses for digressing. Most importantly, you are probably among the majority who are attracted to diets that are of short duration and promise a minimum of discomfort and sacrifice.

The deluge of diet propaganda smothers us in panaceas, and confuses us in contradictions.

Magazine and newspaper editorials and advertisements expound as many methods of taking off weight as there are ways to prepare a pound of ground beef.

They tell you to take off weight by eating all the fat you want and eliminating carbohydrates. Or, stuff yourself with carbohydrates but don't eat fat. You can take off weight by machine, by pills, by hypnosis.

You are told it is possible to lose weight and still eat all you want. That it is ridiculous to deprive yourself of the pleasure of eating baked potatoes with gobs of butter and sour cream, or Eggs Benedict, or a delightful serving of cherry pie à la mode. Have a candy bar when you feel like it. There are so many problems in your life why not indulge yourself with the simple pleasures. After all, there are pills available to compensate for your indulgence. The nostrums for losing weight, available on the market and in the markets, are multiformed and multitudinous.

Have you ever seen anyone more enthusiastic and elated than men or women who have just discovered a new diet or method that is guaranteed to finally put an end to their years of obesity? In almost every instance their enthusiasm is in proportion to the latitude of their diet. The more they are allowed to eat and the less they need to sacrifice, the greater their interest.

I remember an incident at a luncheon with an acquaintance whom I hadn't seen for several years. There was to be a short program before the meal was served, and as is the custom at such times, everyone was served butter and rolls. My companion started telling me about this wonderful weight reducing method which friends of hers had embraced with remarkable results. While she was talking I became completely fascinated watching her eat a pat of butter with a fork. No bread, just the butter. Finally my attention was called back to her conversation and having noticed what must have been amazement, or incredulity, on my face, she quickly explained that she could consume all the butter, as well as other fats she desired, as long as she didn't eat bread with it or a potato under it.

I have no idea how successful this diet was for this woman, but I do know that any success she may have had in losing weight was offset in a poor and even dangerous nutritional practice.

If you are among the many having experienced periods of "dieting binges" you have probably also experienced disappointment in results. Oh, you may have lost some pounds, at least temporarily, but chances are you felt sluggish, irritable, and even depressed. This is the result not of being underfed but undernourished. Many diets, at least the more publicized ones, offer rewards based on privation of important nutrients. The program in this book is founded on the principles of sound nutrition and dietetically prepared menus.

To achieve satisfactory results it is necessary to prepare yourself mentally for it. In this chapter I hope to establish motives to condition you to the most concentrated and healthful effort you have ever exerted to lose those unwanted pounds.

Once you have achieved the desired weight loss and have adjusted your eating habits in accordance with beneficial nutritional patterns, the appeal of highly rich food will diminish.

This results from three factors: (1) a change in thought patterns, (2) a well-nourished body, and (3) the pride in your fitness. Energy lost in obesity will generally be restored in slenderness. Activities you have ignored or avoided will occupy more of your time and thoughts. The obsessions with food will be replaced by useful and beneficial social enterprises.

If you feel you can take off weight without the exercise of willpower and deprivation then set this book down now.

You are overweight because you eat too much, or you eat at the wrong times, or you eat an improper diet, and not because you have inherited obesity. (However, you could well have inherited eating habits that cause your overweight.) It does not come from physical disturbances (only 5 per cent of the obese are thus affected). Compulsion in eating, as in drinking, is not a natural phenomenon but rather a developed one. Our bodies do not "crave" sweets anymore than they "crave" alcohol. The compulsion is created by practice.

I heard a girl lament that she puts on weight merely reading a menu whereas her luncheon campanion can eat anything and everything without losing her shape. Forget it, the eyes do not assimilate calories, but four out of five dishes recommended can be enemies of the obese.

It follows that if you have been overweight a considerable length of time, you have been eating improperly the equivalent length of time.

You have conditioned yourself to live a life of eating food, thinking food and talking food. Even your dreams may include orgies of exotic eating experiences.

Now you must desist from thinking and talking about food. Remove its importance from your life. This is not easy because the American scene is replete with suggestions of delectable menus and recipes. Television commercials, now even more so with the advent of color, offer tempting suggestions, and even in one minute can activate our salivary glands.

Magazines portray exciting delights in beautiful color photography so lifelike we can almost savor the aroma.

As I am writing this, there is appearing in the current issue of one of the largest women's publications, a two-page spread, cleverly prepared, referring to dieting and calories. It includes a 1500 calorie a day program for losing weight. Paradoxically, the two preceeding pages show mouth-watering photographs of a cheese soufflé and apple strudel. The following two pages contain enticing illustrations of ice cream dishes including Pistachio "Layer Cake."

Oh yes, they do refer to recipes to be found far in the back of the magazine that will help you prepare dietary meals. These are not accompanied by photographs, and I defy anyone to read them and erase from memory the strudel and the ice cream delicacies!

To strengthen your determination to lose weight, consider the advantages accruing to a slender body.

HEALTH

Overweight is considered the number one health problem in the United States today, but it isn't a twentieth-century phenomenon. Hippocrates, the Greek physician known as the father of medicine, wrote in 400 B.C., "Fat men are more likely to die suddenly than the slender."

In *Love's Labor's Lost*, Shakespeare considers the effect of obesity on the power of the brain. "Fat paunches have lean pates, and dainty bits make rich the ribs, but bankrupt quite the wits."

Forget the statistic referring to the 50,000,000 Americans who are overweight. At least forget 49,999,999 of them. Dieting is a personal project. I can give you the program, but the motivation must come from you.

Forget the unsuccessful attempts you have made previously. Forget the successful attempts when you took off weight only to replace it with a like amount. (Chances are you have become heavier than you were before the abortive attempt.) Medically, there is evidence that fluctuations in weight, brought about by the periodic use of "fad" diets, may be more damaging to health than a constant state of moderate overweight.

Forget the ingredients, principles and promises of those other diets. They were unsatisfactory or this book wouldn't be of interest to you.

COMFORT

You don't have to admit to being uncomfortable, you look it. Stairs are fearsome, hot weather deplorable, tying shoe laces a chore. Getting in and out of a car is laborious. It isn't a matter of being able to touch your toes, it's a matter of being able to see them.

Walking is uncomfortable, but so is sitting. The simple duties of home care are a burden. Clothes don't fit, nor does even your finest dress or suit made to your present measurements feel comfortable.

APPEARANCE

Look at yourself objectively, other people do. We have lived with our own image so long we are not aware of it.

Test your appearance by glancing in store windows as you shop. View your body in the nude in front of your bedroom mirror. No one has to *tell* you you are overweight. The admission of obesity is essential before you can be convinced you want to lose weight.

PRIDE

A man or woman without pride has little else to compensate for it. Slovenly habits make us dislike ourselves. We are slovenly, or careless, because of a lack. A lack of love, a lack of ambition, a lack of energy, a lack of incentive, a lack of initiative. Somewhere, somehow, we have lost the desire to be admired.

If you find an application of any of these lacks to yourself, then it is important to analyze the reason behind it.

Remember how you looked and felt before you added the unwanted poundage. Do you still have a dress in the closet, or a pair of slacks, or a photograph, that reminds you of your other self, the self you left when the pounds began accumulating? How many years has it been—be honest—since you could slip into your wedding gown, Mrs., or you, Mr., joined a Veterans Day parade in your old uniform? Have you looked at the worn notches in your belt— where it *used* to fit? Do you remember the days on the beach when you didn't want to cover yourself with a towel to hide your shape? Or, have you even stopped going to the beach altogether?

The satisfaction of an attractive figure can be more than gratification of ego. It is an expression of well-adjusted maturity.

Most people need a strong and vivid reason to lose weight. The will power and the privations required to lose weight and keep it off is easier to tolerate if you give yourself an important incentive. But isn't this true with anything worthwhile accomplishing in life?

A young patient of mine had a powerful motive. Married only four years she had gained so much weight she could no longer wear her wedding ring. This was a very emotional experience for her. It was the incentive she needed. When, after a period of some weeks, she was able once more to fit her ring on her finger, she invited friends in and the highlight of the evening was a mock wedding, with her husband slipping the ring on her now slender finger.

This was her motive. What about *you*? If you can't convince yourself that health reasons are strong enough, then consider your appearance, or your pride, or your comfort.

A boy friend or a husband, a girl friend or a wife, might be the reason. Regardless, make sure that you *have* a reason, because it will be of considerable help in the weeks ahead.

Losing weight is a form of self-improvement, just as is learning a foreign language, studying the opera, or joining a great books seminar.

If men would apply themselves as studiously in taking off weight as they do increasing their bowling averages, or studying their trade papers; if women were as conscientious about their diets as they are about their bridge game, or their social obligations, we would be a nation of sveltes instead of swells.

One of the most gratifying by-products of a sensible weight loss is the years that seem to drop from the face. A frequently heard comment from the people I have worked with on the program concerns the effect it has had on their facial appearance. They happily report that their family and friends seem surprised they have not only lost pounds but also years. This is to be expected and not surprising in the least. Weight adds years and therefore it follows that the reduction in weight through a proper nutritional program should take off years. Generally, another contributing factor is the healthy appearance of the complexion. Many of the foods that obese people choose are those that have a negative influence on the complexion. Nourishing foods can put a rose on your cheek, and in many cases, remove blemishes caused by improper diets.

There is an important psychological influence that often reflects itself in the face. People are generally unhappy with their extra poundage and slenderness will bring smiles back, and a smiling face looks more youthful. Also, you are more healthy when you are at your proper weight and a healthy body reflects favorably on your countenance.

The effect of crash diets, or starvation diets, will react unfavorably, leaving you haggard and wan. There is a man in our neighborhood who periodically fights his weight problem with diet binges. His wife actually discourages his participation in these excursions into slenderness because he ends up looking as though he had been ill.

If you apply the precepts in this book you will take off weight for the last time, because you will never again be fat.

2

Parting Is Such Sweet Sorrow

You realize you must lose weight for any or all of the previously discussed advantages of a slender body. You know of no medical reason to prohibit a diet. Regular physical examinations are sensible and of importance—particularly after we have passed the age of thirty.

You *know* you are overweight without consulting a chart. Nevertheless, for a guide, we are including the Metropolitan Life Insurance Company's chart for both men and women in Appendix I.

Next, prepare your own progress chart, a sample to serve as a guide will be found in Appendix II.

Write in the upper left hand corner the date you are starting and your current weight. Remember, when you weigh yourself, it must be at the same time of the day, and preferably in the nude.

Weigh yourself the day you start and then only once a week thereafter. The program is a sound and clinically

tested method of certainty, but not with miraculous over-
night results.

Weighing daily may make you overconfident and result
in lack of diligence. You could decline four or five pounds
in one or two days but this could be the reduction in body
fluids and not a sustained loss. Or, you may go several days
without a loss and thus suffer discouragement.

In the area indicated on the chart, write down your
measurements: upper arms, bust, rib cage, waist, stomach,
hips, thighs, ankles. To prepare for this obtain a reliable
tape measure and keep it handy. You will be using it for
the duration. Remember, you are going to lose weight
where you want to and thus the tape is as important as your
scales.

When you promised yourself to lose weight you did not
do it with reservations. That is, you did not include exceptions in your resolution such as holiday seasons, vacations,
or the many other occasions such as birthdays (in a large
family, or broad social group, these could occur with
regularity), anniversaries, or "I feel sorry for myself"
periods when indulgence seems pacifying.

Don't wait to start the program when the future does not
promise anything unusual to deter your progress. Believe
me when I say there is no better time to start than right
now. With delays, your purpose and determination will
falter and all your promises will dim with time.

If the road to perdition is paved with good intentions,
then alibis are the materials from which the pavement is
formed.

Alibis are used to cover sins of commission or omission
and no more creativity is expended in any one form than
the alibis created to excuse or explain a person's obesity.

Alibis go back two generations to the indulgence of
grandparents who insisted stoutness in children was evidence of health. They include mother whose cooking was

irresistible; father because he harassed them to clean their plate; teachers supervising school lunches and reporting to parents any timidity in eating habits.

Alibis multiply with the approaching starting date of a self-imposed diet. Holidays are coming up . . . a special dinner party . . . birthday . . . "I feel a little peaked and best keep up my strength" . . . "I won't be able to wear my new dress to the dance next month" . . . "My vacation begins next week."

You want to be slender and stay slender. Not a year from now, but as soon as this dietetic program will allow. You may be the fortunate minority who require a loss of only 8 to 10 pounds. Fortunate, yes, because you can accomplish your goal sooner, but my experience has shown that men and women with 30 or 40 or more pounds of excess weight will demonstrate considerably more determination than those who are only a relatively few pounds away from a slender, lithe figure.

Procrastination not only leads to a longer period of obesity, but during the delay most people will add additional pounds because, "I'll take them all off when I start next week."

A program of weight reduction based on sound nutritional practices does not allow the transgression of the fad diets where today's sins can be absolved by tomorrow's penitence.

Like any of our living patterns and habits, this program is easier to follow if you make it a part of a daily regimen. Exceptions only make it more difficult. Indulging yourself with a chocolate éclair this afternoon is not going to make tomorrow's diet routine easier. But, each time you overcome the temptation of a forbidden tidbit you will find resistance easier the next time. It is no different than the repulsion of any temptation. Your conscience and deportment is strengthened with application of willpower, whether it be to stop smoking, exercise regularly, or follow a diet. You are doing it for your own good. You aren't cheating on your doctor or me, you are cheating yourself—cheating yourself of all the delights and benefits that derive from a slender body.

In *The Life of Samuel Johnson* by James Boswell, we read, "Some people have a foolish way of not minding, or pretending not to mind, what they eat. For my part, I mind my belly very studiously and very carefully, for I look upon it that he who does not mind his belly will hardly mind anything else."

That could pretty well sum up what dietetics and nutrition is all about. To eliminate all the fancy phrases and definitions, we are only talking about what to put in your stomach to make you healthy and restore a youthful energetic shape to a body you have neglected through overindulgence and lack of nutritional care. It is a sign of intelligence, as well as maturity, to take care of your body.

The promises I make in this book are based on reciprocation. You follow the precepts and I promise you a slender and attractive body for the rest of your life. Furthermore, I promise you will look younger, feel better, be more energetic and healthier.

Are these results sufficient compensation for what may appear to you now as sensual satisfactions? I say, appear to you *now*, because it has been my experience with the great majority of obese men and women I have worked with that food obsession gradually diminishes and pride of accomplishment replaces it.

Remove temptation from your mind as well as your reach.

I have heard people who have stopped smoking say it strengthened their resolve to smell cigarette smoke or even pick one up in their hands, going as far as putting it in their mouths. Whether this is a form of masochism I do not know, but I have never found this method of deliberate temptation to work in dieting.

Men have been heard to complain that when their wives go on diets the only ones to lose weight were themselves. This implies the imposition of a regimentation upon the innocent. The "misery loves company" thinking. It will help to remember when your doctor has prescribed medicine for you, you didn't make other members of your family take it.

Preparing meals in accordance with a prescribed diet for your husband should be undertaken with the same thoughtfulness and consideration as you would display in eliminating sweets from his diet if he were a diabetic. Overweight is a medically accepted health hazard and many more people expire from the multiple effects of obesity than from diabetes. And just as diabetes can be controlled, so can obesity.

If it is the woman of the house that is the subject of a diet then she should make it a personal thing and restrict its obligations to herself. I realize this may mean cooking, smelling, and seeing forbidden delights day after day. However, there are many delicious and even gourmet items, recipes and menus available within your diet. Ingenuity is an important ingredient in any menu planning, and the application of ingenuity in diet menus can result in an appetizing variety of dishes.

Your personal privation must not be imposed upon the other members of the family for one very sound reason— happiness. It is important to you and your family that tranquility not be jeopardized. Any disturbance caused by a dieting man or woman in a home could greatly increase the possibility of either a cessation of the program or at least detrimental compromises and modifications.

Later I will discuss the reasons for not talking indiscriminately about your diet with other people, but this does not apply entirely to other members of your household. At the outset explain what you are going to do and why. The love and mutual consideration in a family will pave the way for a successful and gratifying program. After this initial discussion, refrain from talking about it even to your family.

Breaking a habit will not be made easier by my saying you must use all the resources of your willpower. The U. S. Surgeon General's Report on the effects of cigarette smoking did not result in any appreciable decline in the dissemination of the habit. My telling you of the program's benefits can only be an encouragement. In Chapter 12 I report a number of case histories from my clinic. They are included in this book as a demonstration of the program's effectiveness, but every bit as important is the help it may be to you in pursuit of a trim body.

3

Sex by the Pound

Since the enlightenment inspired and promulgated by Freud on the importance and power of the human sex drive, the subject has emerged from the alleys and has extended beyond the snickers of young sophisticates. Having been acknowledged as a normal, God-given urge, it is now freely discussed as the basis for many psychological disturbances. In no area does its influence have greater significance than in obesity.

Children will sometimes develop abnormal eating patterns due to lack of demonstrated affection by a parent. This same parent can be influenced to a similar eating pattern, due to sexual neglect.

More frequently, however, as recorded in my case-history files, are instances of diminished connubial intimacy resulting from the unattractiveness produced by obesity.

A female patient who had successfully completed the program with a net loss of 32 pounds reported that her two daughters, ages twenty-one and nineteen, observed, "Daddy acts so much more amorously toward you since your weight loss."

Another women, after six weeks on the program, brought her husband with her on one of her visits. His comment was, "I feel as though I have my bride back."

Obesity can lead to the lack of desire. Even as stairs become more difficult to climb so do amorous pursuits. A thirty-seven year old man, 5'9", who had reduced from 220 pounds to 182 confessed it wasn't his wife who had lost interest in him. "I would fall asleep in a chair after dinner and later arouse myself just enough to put on my pajamas and climb into bed to continue sleeping. Sex wasn't the only thing I lost interest in," he continued, "I quit playing golf."

A husband will start to compare his overweight wife with the slender figures in his office, or the girls he observes on the bus. He remembers the way his wife looked during their courtship days. Frequently he will take her neglect and carelessness as a personal slight.

This neglect is reflected in other than her appearance. As her weight increases, her energy decreases. The greater the weight, the more difficult becomes the routine efforts of maintaining a home. Tiredness accompanies obesity and more hours are spent napping or sitting. Listlessness replaces vivaciousness, and inertia replaces previously shared family activities.

Recently, a girl of seventeen came to my office for her first visit. As is my custom, I attempted to establish a reason for her weight concern in the initial interview. Once the reason (or reasons) is established I use this as the motivation for faithful adherence to the program. Sometimes patients are reluctant to reveal their *true* reason during the first session. Generally, however, they will blurt it out within a few minutes; often with what seems great relief in expressing what they have kept suppressed.

This girl, whom I will give the name Suzy (all names

used in this book are, of course, fictitious for professional and courtesy reasons), seemed anxious to talk and a rapport was easily established.

A junior in high school, Suzy has never had a date with a boy—"not even a coke date, Mrs. Boody," was her lament. Now perhaps when some of us were her age it wasn't the custom for *every* girl to date, but among the changes in times are those involving the boy–girl relationship. The average, first-time, marriage age has lowered eight years since the end of World War II. More girls marry before twenty than marry later. More girls marry at eighteen than any other age.

Suzy has an amazingly clear, unblemished complexion. Her eyes are deep brown and her hair shows evidence of careful, thoughtful grooming. She is 5'5" tall. She also weighs 178 pounds.

"I used to console myself with the thought that I was too young to date," she said as her eyes began to glisten with emotion. "I was told at home it was baby fat and would dissolve with maturity."

I have never been more confident in the ultimate success of a patient than I am with Suzy. She has the strongest motivation for leaving the ranks of the obese—sex!

A woman who had completed the program three years previously called for an appointment. After our phone conversation, assuming she had retrogressed, I looked up her file. She had lost 52 pounds with her bust measurement decreasing from 50 to 39 inches—her hips from 52 to 40 inches. There were two photographs in the file—a before and an after. Do you suppose, I wondered, after these marvelous results she returned to obesity? This has not happened often to those on this program, but circumstances in a person's life will sometimes cause them to revert to old patterns.

With these thoughts in mind, I was pleased to see her as I last did, slender and lovely. Following her was a young boy, looking much like the son of the woman in the before photograph.

"This is George," she said by way of introduction, "and he has agreed to try the program." After they left, she returned to my office a moment later, alone. "You may not remember, but three years ago," she said, "I tried to get George interested in taking off weight. I had hopes that my success would encourage him, but nothing helped. Instead, he continued to gain."

"Now," she continued, "he is sixteen. All his friends are dating girls and the only girl that seems to be the least bit interested in him is one with a similar weight problem. He finds her unattractive and so doesn't date at all. Finally, the frankness of youth expressed itself. His friends told him he would never get a girl because he is too fat."

The desire to be admired and desired by the opposite sex is as consistent with normality as breathing and sleeping and the need of nourishment.

Wall flowers are not the lithe, lovely, slender, long-stem American Beauties. They are the bulky, heavy leafed *Taraxacum* (dandelion, that is).

The beach bully really *didn't* kick sand in the face of a skinny kid. He could have at least defended himself by running away. It was a fat blubbery guy, who would have a problem of lifting himself off the sand, let alone sprinting out of danger.

The great lovers of history do not include the gross Henry VIII, in spite of myth. The courtesans of the eighteenth century wore wide, bulky bustles but there was considerably less beneath the surface than met the eye.

The thick neck and vast girth may still be the prototype of a truck driver, but J. P. Morgan's proportions no longer fit today's financiers.

Opulence is no longer measured by corpulence.

And whatever sexual symbol may have been expressed in the "beef trust" of early vaudeville has been replaced by the slender loveliness of today's chorus girl.

The "heavy" in Hollywood's vernacular may be just that; however, seldom does he win the girl.

The sex symbol was expressed by Rubens as a buxom, heavy-thighed, round-bottomed lass; but that was in the seventeenth century. Today the proportions are those of the sylphlike nymph gracing the pages of our fashion pages and television screens.

Two out of three people seeking help in my clinic are concerned with the effect of obesity on their love life. Young girls, like Suzy, who can't seem to find a social life involving boys; men who have been frustrated in their attempts to find the "right girl"; married women who have realized a noticeable "lack of interest" on the part of their husband; even children of fourteen and fifteen have been directed to me by their parents because they seem to have no energy, no desire of participation, and lack companionship.

Men are the most reluctant to seek professional help—perhaps because of that esoteric "male ego."

Strangely—and to most of us women, mystifying—is the male attitude that obesity in women is deplorable, whereas in men it's acceptable.

If a fat woman is unattractive to the man, let me assure you male readers that the complaints I hear from female patients give you overweight "tigers" the sexual reputation of "kittens."

Inertia follows rapidly in the path of obesity. Think of years when the "chase" was as rewarding as the conquest. Every ten pounds you've added has diminished proportionately the desire for either.

Think of your personal criterion for dreams of romance.

Do you, a woman, visualize a man of Falstaffian proportions? Do you, a man, picture companionship with a woman whose girth is greater than your reach?

A woman patient, I'll call Madge, had been married twelve years when she had her first child. The joy and ecstasy experienced by her and her husband were unbounded, she explained. They had wanted children all these years and had suffered the denial including three early miscarriages.

Compensation for the lack of children they found in a strong mutual love. "We had each other," Madge added, "and if God saw fit to restrict our family to the two of us, we would be eternally grateful for the love we shared."

Now, Madge said, she not only seriously questioned her husband's love, but his fidelity. The child was eighteen months old and Madge admitted to weighing, at the time of our first interview, seven pounds more than prior to delivery.

"Ed was on a cloud for months," she said, "then gradually he was later and later getting home. I gave up being annoyed because with my slightest criticism he became so irritated he would leave the house for the entire evening."

Finally Madge admitted to herself that the blame was hers. Not because she lavished affections on the child to the neglect of her husband, but because her fulfillment as a mother and devotion to her daughter and the father, made her completely selfless, neglecting herself. While this was being written, Madge was losing sixteen pounds. Her marital problems may not be resolved completely but progress is evident as she reported over the phone: "Ed is taking me to a supper club this evening. I had to call you because the florist just delivered a lovely gardenia corsage."

There is no question, from my experience, that Madge will return to her previous size 8. Her motivation is the strongest—love.

Many are the volumes and articles written on sexual behavior, both scientific and sensational, but the effect of obesity on sex has been virtually ignored. This may be due to obesity being considered a health problem and not a social one. The association between a well-adjusted sex life and overweight may not be generally recognized, but I can assure you it is experienced. Sex is motivated by the stimulation generated by an attraction between man and woman. This is physical, just as obesity is physical. A fat body is not attractive. It violates all the accepted precepts for being appealing, or if you will, sexy.

My reference to sex is not confined to the physical act. A woman with a penchant for looking desirable does not make her wanton. It is normal and healthy for a woman to glow under the admiring glances of men. And men are certainly not impervious to the admiration of women. This has an effect not only on our egoes, but it contributes immeasurably to self-confidence.

A man will take a little more care in the selection of a suit and the choice of a tie when he has an important business meeting, or a significant social engagement. A woman will spend hours in a beauty salon prior to an evening out, or in preparation for entertaining. This is not entirely stimulated by ego. The avidity with which we prepare ourselves for being "viewed" is prompted by a need to feel assured in the company of others. Self-confidence will result in knowing we look our best. Women will buy a new hat or obtain a new coiffure when they are feeling depressed. This acts more as a stimulant to self-confidence than as balm to the ego.

Unfortunately, even the most careful grooming can't hide grossness. Beauty is *not* only skin deep. The deposits of fat beneath the skin can make an otherwise lovely woman or handsome man unattractive. This is not usually considered, because fat men and women aren't observed closely enough to determine if they have beauty. The bulk of the obese will quickly discourage any careful observance. Even beautiful eyes and a handsome profile will be lost in facial fat accumulation.

There is evidence of a correlation between sexual inhibitions and obesity. People will use grossness as a sex repellent. Rather than formulating the strategies of resistance contrived by the sexually attractive, they cloak themselves in layers of fat, thus eliminating themselves from the unwanted attention of the opposite sex. This tactic may be either a conscious or subconscious effort. This drastic evasion is generally successful in repelling, but it contributes nothing toward a solution of their neurosis. Obesity merely leads to additional problems involving health and emotional stresses.

Overweight results as often from careless dietary habits as it does by excessive caloric intake, and thus it frequently expresses itself in poor complexions and lusterless eyes.

Obesity is not only a deterrent to sexual attractiveness and appeal, excessive amounts of fat reduces energy output whether it be to perform on the golf course or in the boudoir.

The ability, as well as the desire, for physical exertion is reduced in ratio to the amount of excess fat deposited on our bodies. This is not psychological, but physiological. Body energy is expended in the movement of unwanted, unneeded and undesired weight.

The sex urge is both primitive and contemporary. It is natural and salubrious. It is also the most successful incentive I have observed in years of treating the obese.

4

The Diet With a Difference

It is important to continually impress upon you that this is a *new* way to lose fat deposits; and thus for ultimate success, it is necessary for you to discard previous notions about dieting. You cannot compromise by combining or including portions of other weight reducing methods.

Happily, you are relieved of the laborious and tedious procedure of counting calories. Also, you are not required to be hungry at any time of the day. In fact, your appetite will be assuaged frequently during the day. I am not eliminating between-meal eating but encouraging it with a schedule of three meals and three "snack" periods each day.

The quantity permitted at any one sitting may be less than your current consumption, however, you are allowed to eat *six times each day*. All food intake is during the periods when your physical activity is at its peak. With smaller amounts of food your body has an opportunity to assimilate your intake without accumulating fat deposits.

I will not go into all the physiological functions resulting in the accumulation of fat. This is a subject for a medical book. My responsibility as a dietitian is to select and prepare foods to perform most efficiently and nutritionally for a healthy, slender and vigorous body. Suffice it to say, the metabolic pattern of the obese is not normal; and proper foods in proper amounts at proper intervals will result in the correction of abnormal metabolism and put you on the road to a healthy, slender physique.

"The fat get fatter and the lean get leaner," may be the lament of the obese, but they are actually closer to the truth than they assume because fat develops fat, and the more fat the body contains the greater capacity it has to produce fat. An obese body forms and stores fat at a higher than normal rate and disposes of it at a lower than normal rate. This program is designed to change this and the change which occurs will help you maintain the weight loss.

A compatibility is created between food chemistry and body chemistry. This process is the reason why you lose weight where you want to—where fat deposits have amassed. Many of my patients are only slightly overweight but have unattractive fat layers on rib cage, waist and buttocks.

Perhaps the most serious criticism of many diets, particularly the "fad" diets and the "quickies," involves the source of the weight loss. Frequently it is lean muscle tissue rather than fat. This causes a haggard look, the way people might look after a long illness. Folds of flesh appear on the neck and wrinkles on the face. This can occur in young people but is more prevalent in those over forty.

The reduction by the method outlined in this book will not produce wrinkles or flesh folds, because the loss is gradual and does not affect muscle tissues.

Another cause for dramatic reduction from other diets is loss of liquid weight. This can occur quickly and will cause much elation; however, this loss is only temporary.

Trying to lose weight solely through exercise is practically impossible. You would have to walk five miles to burn off the energy of a candy bar, or seven miles after consuming a nut-covered ice cream sundae. If you had enough stamina to walk these miles, you would very likely build up an appetite to replace all loss in one sitting. Exercise, however, does have an important place in this program. A simple, easy, and even enjoyable routine that is designed to tone muscles and to stimulate blood flow is included. You will find this practical, ten-minute-a-day, "Top to Toe" conditioning program in Chapter 11.

The rapidity of weight loss, of course, will depend on your present weight and the amount to be removed; however, the average range is from 12 to 18 pounds per month. This is *permanent* loss. The program will instruct you in the kinds and amounts of food to eat as well as establishing a pattern of consumption that will enable you to *always* control your weight.

In addition to the exterior evidence of weight loss there will also be the important loss of fat around the vital organs of your body. This, of course, is not visible, but is perhaps more significant than the effect on vanity.

Normally, results will begin to evidence themselves after two weeks on the program. You will have increased energy and a feeling of well-being. You will sleep better and even look better. This results not only from weight loss, but also from being properly nourished. The food you will be consuming is nutritionally perfect and thus benefits you in all physiological areas.

Your relationship with your family must be considered. Actually your weight adjustment program can be of great benefit to them, because you have gained knowledge of the basics of nutrition and can apply it for the entire family. This does not mean your family need be deprived, but rather adjusted to better eating habits. Let them eat their desserts and other items they enjoy, but are denied you. Don't impose denials on them—only benefits.

It is important that you talk as little as possible about your dieting to family, friends and acquaintances. Well-meaning friends will make it more difficult for you by suggesting "a little bit won't hurt," or by telling about their favorite diet or suggesting "rest periods" from the regimentation. This is your personal effort and temptations offered you—even with the best of intentions—could set you back in the program, thus causing not only a time loss but possible discouragement.

People do not generally watch what others eat unless their attention has been directed to it. Therefore, by not discussing your crusade, comments can be avoided. When the menu—either in a restaurant or in a home—does not offer your requirements, merely avoid the worse offenders and eat lightly of the others.

Remember, for encouragement at the early stages of the program, although your weight loss will be permanent, you will not have to live a life of perpetual privation. When you have reached the desired level of weight and your metabolism is compatible with your intake, you can go back to a more diversified diet. Your compulsion to overeat will gradually diminish in intensity and eventually disappear. Also, the successful conclusion of the program will result in such gratifying rewards that you will have no desire to return to the old ways.

Weigh yourself once a week, at the same time of the day. At this time take your measurements, noting the figures on the chart you have prepared from the example in Appendix II. Measurements should always be taken in the nude. This is also true when weighing.

You may notice some weeks that you have had little weight loss but noticeable changes in measurements. This is caused by the reduction in fat formations, reducing your areas of obesity and at the same time a retention of water causing a retention of weight. Physiologically what is taking place is the oxidation of fat, resulting in metabolic water.

In the beginning you may also show decreases in upper body measurements but slight increases in legs and ankles. This again is water retention and no cause for alarm. The slight swelling will disappear in a short time.

Early in the book I told you the program was a personal one and that in order to embark on it and sustain it, you need motivation and self-discipline. If there is no evidence of weight loss and changes in measurements then I can assure you from experience with hundreds of cases that you are not following the program or else are allowing yourself an occasional indulgence. Until you have decreased to your proper weight, even small compromises in the program will trigger fat laydown.

It is important that you not only change your eating patterns but also your thought patterns. Overweight people invariably spend a great amount of time thinking about food, planning menus, studying recipes, browsing through food markets, pastry shops and candy stores. Try replacing these thoughts and activities, whenever they occur, with thoughts about the last movie you saw; or pick up a book and read. Try to replace food obsessions with other interests: art, music, a lunch time walk. This may not be easy to do in the beginning, but you will find as time goes by you have many more interesting diversions than food. Keeping food out of your thoughts will keep it out of your mouth.

5

Be Kind to the Kids

A parent's primary concern is for the happiness and well-being of their offspring. In the pursuit of being a good and conscientious mother or father, a great deal of thought, money and effort is expended in making certain their children are well-dressed, well-educated and well-entertained. No sacrifice is too great to see that Susie gets dancing lessons and Johnny goes to camp.

Vacations are planned around the children. Couples with small youngsters arrange their social activities to suit the availability of the most reliable baby-sitters. Families making a move to a new neighborhood or town search first for the best schools and then select a house convenient to the school.

The youth market is a primary target in the marketing objectives of many corporations. Magazines for the young are a major publishing force and are designed for the purpose of reaching youth in an atmosphere created for merchandising products attractive to them. Cosmetics, an industry not so long ago devoted to adult women, now spend astronomical sums in wooing the teenagers, who are reported to spend twenty-two cents of every cosmetic dollar.

I am not going to criticise this twentieth-century fever for pampering and indulging the young. My qualifications for doing so do not exceed the millions of other mothers in the country. My concern is dietetics and thus I am going to direct my words to the nutritional well-being of your children.

My reason for including this chapter is based on this love we demonstrate in so many ways and yet contradict by lack of dietary supervision. Those of you who have suffered the ignominy of obesity through overeating and poor diets should be the first to want to spare your children a similar fate.

A plump baby is a status symbol. It signifies the adequacy of the mother. When normal growth changes the appearance of a round baby to a slim child, the parent's concern will result in an effort to put "meat on those bones." As a child leaves babyhood and enters childhood the importance of food diminishes, and the appetite is depressed. This will often result in parental anxiety and can trigger an overemphasis on eating that will result in the eventual fat child.

In a well-organized household, with thoughtfulness and care used in the preparation of well-balanced meals, it is impossible for a child to suffer from malnutrition. In the course of growing up he or she will adapt to an orderly diet. Guidance by the parent is, of course, essential because the habits and feeding patterns of the parents are highly influential in determining the child's own eating program. Force-feeding of the child will generally become a long-term endeavor resulting in the offspring joining the ranks of the obese.

Bad habits need not be overcome if they are never formed, and in no area is this more true than in the development of eating patterns. Healthful nutritional habits formed when young will contribute more to future happiness than a dance class or a new rocket toy. A well-balanced diet and thoughtful menus contribute to the general health and growth of the child. This does not mean making up deficiencies with vitamin pills.

Food selection and preferences develop when we are very young, and guidance in proper eating habits is the responsibility of the parents. Many are the people I have seen whose problems originated while they were young and under parental supervision. The habit of eating more than the body requires is one of the most frequent violations. Indiscriminate snacking, or the open-door policy (refrigerator door, that is), is not a demonstration of love.

Fat children suffer when they reach the age of socializing on a broader level, such as school. The slights and hurts experienced by the obese child are hardly worth the indulgence that caused them; and this includes only the obvious and not what might be impairment of health.

It is normal for active children to get hungry between meals and they should be nourished at that time—note that I said *nourished*. A glass of milk, a slice of cheese, some fruit—these contribute to their well-being. An occasional piece of candy, bottle of pop, a dish of ice cream, is certainly not objectionable. A high school student who has never visited the "malt shop" hasn't completed his education. These simple pleasures are not what I am referring to —I am referring to the constant nibbling of candy, washed down by magnums of sweet drinks, and the habit of demanding something to eat prior to a meal, resulting in lack of appetite at the important feeding periods.

The most effective way to create desirable traits in children is by example—the example of the parents. You begin early to develop their table manners and are even more careful than usual with your own deportment at the table when the children are present. Be equally concerned with the dietary example you set. Here are a few suggestions you might find useful:

1. Make healthful nourishing foods available. This means the preparation of good nutritious meals, and the accessibility of beneficial snacks.

2. Milk is still considered, by most, as the world's "most perfect food." The vitamins, minerals and protein make it so. Full fat milk will not hurt a child that does not tend toward heaviness, but remember, skim milk or low-fat milk retains all the important elements with only the butterfat removed or reduced. Milk continues to be beneficial to us all of our lives. We do not outgrow the need for milk, only the desire. Unless you are among the very few to whom milk is intolerable, set an example by serving *all* the family a glass of milk at dinner time. Don't try to pass off your lack of interest in milk by claiming it is "for children." Children love to emulate their parents. They don't want to eat children's food; they want to eat adult food. This is why coffee is so fascinating to the young.

3. Try to prevent your child from "specializing" in food. If left to their own preference, children will often concentrate on one or two items. Sometimes it is meat, sometimes it is mashed potatoes, and other times the only satisfying diet is bread with any number of assorted coatings. It is true they grow out of this eating pattern, but it is not necessary for it to become established in the first place. Make available on their plates an assortment of foods. Do not leave them to their own devices in selecting their own specialties if they show such an inclination. If either of the parents does not like broccoli, don't serve it rather than have your children observe your distaste. If a child con-

sistantly resists a particular vegetable don't try to force it upon him. The year-around availability of a great variety of vegetables leaves no excuse for not allowing a choice. Most vegetables contain the same food values and therefore if your family prefers green beans, cauliflower, asparagus and Brussels sprouts, they will lack nothing nutritionally if they concentrate on these.

4. Try new foods and new preparation of old favorites. There are so many rewards in the future of a child if they develop a taste for exciting dishes. Do I sound inconsistent? On the one hand teaching careful eating habits to avoid overweight and then suggesting you make gourmets out of your children? Not at all. Being a gourmet does not make a person overweight. There are as many slender gourmets as there are fat ones. A gourmet is a connoisseur in eating— a gourmand is one who eats excessively. It is the selection and the quantity that separates the two.

5. The importance of a nourishing breakfast has been propounded by medical authorities and dietitians through every means of communication and with every possible argument. I can add no more, except to emphasize the importance of the adults in the home setting the example for the young by eating sensibly in the morning.

6. Earlier in the book I mentioned that a considerable number of obesity cases originate as children through parents who consider quantity as nourishment. These children have the most difficult time in losing weight in later years. Habits created early are the most difficult to break. Be concerned about *what* your child eats and the quantity will generally take care of itself. Psychologists seem to agree that obesity in children results from: (a) having an excessive amount of food pressed upon them, (b) overeating to compensate for a lack of love and affection, or (c) following the example of parents who overeat. If you, the parent, eat carefully and sensibly you are not only help-

ing yourself, but the entire family. Maybe this is even a
stronger incentive and motive than those we discussed
previously.

It is hoped that the truths learned in this book concerning
the disadvantages of obesity and how it can be resolved
through proper nutrition and sensible eating patterns will
also benefit your children and your husband or wife. Health
is a family project and good eating habits are necessary for
good health and a happy coexistence.

6

Tips for Tots and Teenagers

As a guide to help young people stay slender, or remove weight if they are beginning to get "chubby," I am enumerating some practices which have proved to be successful. You will note they are based on common sense and do not include magic formulas, or difficult and tedious regimentation.

This advice is not meant to inhibit youthful pleasures and activities, but rather to make life more enjoyable during the happy young years. Sensible nutritional habits will supply the energy needed to participate in sports and social activities with zest.

If, of course, the child is obviously overweight, the diet presented in this book should be used. The following suggestions will then enable him or her to maintain the weight loss following the conclusion of the diet.

DO

Eat Slowly

This aids digestion and helps prevent overeating.

Eat Smaller Portions of a Greater Variety of Food

Our bodies require the nutrients found in an assortment of foods such as meat, vegetables, fish, fruits and cereals.

Drink Diet Pop

This makes an ideal snack because it is sweet, filling and yet not fattening.

Eat Breakfast Every Day

This is an important meal because it comes at the time of day when you begin your energetic activities.

Eat Only One Large Meal a Day

If, as is generally the case, your main meal is dinner, then go light at lunch.

Walk More

I say "more" because in today's society it can be assumed you don't walk enough. Walking is one of the most beneficial exercises and the simplest to do. If you must ride —do it on a bicycle.

Exercise

Lazy children are frequently fat children. Exercising will make you hungry but it will also burn up calories and make your body firm and more attractive. It might be encouraging to know that dancing is good exercise.

DON'T

Eat Dessert With Your Meal

If you wish a dessert, save it for a mid-afternoon or evening snack.

Be a Bore

If you place yourself on a diet make it a personal thing and don't inflict it on your friends—unless a friend volunteers to join you. Having a companion in the effort can strengthen your resolve.

Lose Too Much Too Fast

The best diets are those that take weight off gradually. This weight loss will be more easily maintained. Also, if you try to take off weight quickly your energy output can suffer and you might become listless and irritable.

Let Your Social Life Suffer

Make it easy on yourself. If you wish to take off weight don't deprive yourself of fun activities while you are doing it. Be intelligent about your intake and your body will take care of the rest.

Eliminate All "Fun" Foods

Rather than abstaining from all foods that are fattening, merely cut down on amounts and frequency. Eat ice cream without the sauce and nuts. Eat only one-half an order of french fries. Drink diet pop rather than those rich in sugar.

Rely on Pills

Weight reducing pills frequently result in nervousness and even illness. If you want to remain slender, eat sensibly. If you have weight you want removed, follow the program in this book.

BE HIP—NOT HIPPY

7

Thin Thoughts

It became evident to me years ago: people with a weight problem also have a thought problem. The propensity for food has its origin in the mind. The stomach might signal the need for food, but frequently the need is initiated by thought processes. A man once told me he never paid any attention to the clock while at work, and when lunch time came around he wasn't prepared to eat. "However," he added, "when I sit in a restaurant and read the menu I get ravishing." His mind, rather than the stomach cravings generally associated with hunger, is telling him he is hungry.

Invariably, men and women I have advised in an eating program will ask how they can break a lifelong habit of thinking about food. My suggestion is thought substitution. That is why, in weight therapy, we recommend the subject engage in activities disassociated with food. The salivary glands do not operate independently—they are stimulated by mental images. By avoiding thoughts of food the yearning can be greatly reduced. The mind controls the body including the stomach. This is not to imply that there is no physical indication of hunger. No one can say the "growl-ings" of a demanding stomach are imaginary, however; even these can be stimulated by our thoughts.

Analyze your own hunger patterns. Chances are you will admit to most food longings in periods of boredom, or at least, inactivity. Often I hear people say their greatest period of food obsession is in the evening. Even cautious eating during the day can be dissipated with indulgence at night. Activities of the day behind them, a few hours of relaxation in front of the television set and then begins the craving for additional food. It "gives me something to do," is a frequent explanation.

Nibbling can be a reflex, similar to smoking. Perhaps you have admitted, if you smoke cigarettes, that many of those you smoke are lighted without a conscious act. This seems to be a common pattern and can also be associated with eating. Many people admit to picking up a piece of candy, a cookie, or a slice of cake and eating it without being com-pletely aware they were doing so. Habits follow a pattern of reflexes, and these habits can be controlled only by will of the mind.

I have counseled men and women who actually cannot tell me their daily consumption—even when I refer to yesterday. From experience, I know they are not being evasive. They honestly do not recall each morsel they have eaten. To help them understand the reason for their obesity I will request that they write down everything they consume in a day. The volume and frequency of feeding many times comes as a surprise even to themselves.

The admission of compulsive eating is an important step in the final solution. When evasion is detected I refer to the interest they have in the program. It is necessary to be honest with themselves before they can honestly follow this program or any program of self-improvement.

A major effort in working with the obese is the determination of the reason or reasons for their overweight. Most often it has a foundation of psychological significance. By the time they come to me they have generally recognized their problem and are prepared to meet the requirements demanded in the program. Those who are not mentally adjusted to a reducing program have far greater difficulty in pursuing the program successfully.

There are many tricks the obese use in disguising their eating habits, even from themselves. A woman will refer to the conservative amount of food she consumes at a meal, and ignore the tasting that accompanied the preparation. Or, they refuse to acknowledge the number of snacks they consume in a day.

One woman, who insisted she ate sparingly at meal time, finally admitted to a practice that removed any doubts about her source of weight. She had three young children who followed a not unfamilar pattern of leaving food on their plates. Detesting waste of any nature she would clean their plates for them rather than "throw good food out." She added, "I was told repeatedly, by my mother when I was a child, that if I wasted food I would some day go hungry."

It is a sad paradox that in many parts of the world, people by the millions do not get enough to eat, and in the affluent nations people by the millions get too much to eat. But we do not help the starving people by developing a neurosis of the "clean plate" in our children. It is a far worse offense to force food youngsters at an early age and then watch them grow into obese teenagers and adults than it is to "waste" the little food they may leave. A simple solution is to put less food on their plates. Many children will lose their appetite if too much is placed before them. Give them smaller amounts and let them ask for more if they remain hungry.

Men will keep bags of candy or salted nuts in their desk drawers at the office. "Just a little something to tide me over," is the excuse. They will then display a virtuous mien

at the luncheon table with companions by eating lightly
and adding a sugar substitute to their coffee.

Overweight people are quick to state that they eat no
breakfast, as though this were a matter of pride, rather
than a ridiculous and harmful eating pattern. For some
reason, which is a little difficult to explain, most overweight people do not eat breakfast.

Some of the most severe cases of obesity espouse the
following eating pattern: no breakfast, snack type lunch
and a moderate-size dinner followed by constant snacking
until bed time. During their active daytime hours, when
nourishment is required for energy, they fast. This results
in their using up lean muscle tissue for energy. The nighttime feedings therefore turn to additional fat.

The program in this book requires frequent feedings
(six) during the daytime hours when the food is allowed
to be burned up in energy. This not only prevents fat accumulation, but nourishes the body in order to provide
energy for our normal activities.

Extensive research has been done on the effect of fasting
during the day and "making up for it" at night. In one
study it was found that on the same number of calories,
fat accumulated twenty-five times faster with concentrated
nighttime feeding.

This erratic eating is the result of thought patterns. First
of all, these people will reason—and often rightfully—that
they are not consuming excessive amounts in a total day.
Secondly, their minds are occupied with numerous diversions during the day. When night comes, and it is time to
relax, their mind becomes obsessed with food and thus
begins the restless pacing back and forth to the refrigerator and candy dish and pastry box.

All too often this feeding process does not conclude with
retiring, as many will get up in the middle of the night and
continue snacking. Doesn't it stand to reason food con-
sumed during inactive hours will be retained? You are not

expending energy during these periods, and thus it offers an excellent opportunity for your body chemistry to develop additional fat deposits.

Only you have control over your thoughts. I cannot make you think thin thoughts; however, I can offer some suggestions that have been helpful to others.

1. Make food as unavailable as possible. Don't leave bonbons and nuts in accessible dishes. Try to avoid having tempting snacks handy.

2. Upon awakening in the morning, adjust your thoughts to the appetizing breakfast outlined in the program. This is *not* the time to avoid thinking about food.

3. If nibbling seems irresistible in the evening and you have trouble keeping your thoughts off the temptation, try taking a walk, or a relaxing warm bath.

4. If the evening snack—as recommended in the program—does not satisfy you, drink a glass of diet pop just before retiring.

5. Keep your mind as free of food as possible. Until your mind has been conditioned to resist tantalizing images of food you should avoid tormenting yourself by looking at the magnificent photographs found in magazine food editorials and advertisements.

6. Think about the reasons you are on a weight reducing program. Whenever food images begin to crowd your mind, make a concentrated effort to drive them out with thoughts involving the motivations we have discussed in Chapter 1 or Chapter 3. Thought patterns are no easier to change than eating patterns and so I advise you to reread Chapter 1 as often as is necessary to strengthen your resolve.

With each day of faithfulness to the program, the next day's effort will be a little less tedious. The encouragement you receive as your weight drops, and your measurements reflect the loss, will be a strong influence on your thought processes. Temptations will become easier and easier to resist.

8

Fantasies, Fallacies, Facts About Food

Down through recorded history, as well as in mythology, are reported taboos, superstitions and religious restrictions concerning the consumption, and in some instances, the preparation of food.

Fanaticism in some countries has resulted in widespread malnutrition and even starvation while the land offers them, if not abundance, sufficiency.

Superstition encouraged by ignorance, old wives' tales supported by tradition, have had a part in disseminating misinformation about food and its function.

Even in our well-informed society there are a great many erroneous concepts involving even the most common of foods.

As an example, milk. There is a widespread belief that milk is a child's food and is not beneficial, and is even perhaps harmful, to the adult. Milk is an economical source of high-quality protein, calcium, and the vitamin riboflavin. These nutrients are required at any age, and doctors frequently include milk in special diets because it is easily digested. There also exists the mistaken belief that pasteurized milk contains less nutritive value than raw milk. There is an overwhelming amount of evidence that pasteurized milk will result in the same rate of growth in children as will raw milk. The possibility of diseases contracted from raw milk should make pasteurization compulsory everywhere.

The acid from oranges is sometimes considered detrimental to those suffering from rheumatism. Actually the acid from fruit is converted to a base which neutralizes acids from other sources that are harmful to the rheumatic.

Whole wheat bread is held to be an important substitute for white bread. While whole wheat bread does have better nutritive values than white, these are not significant because the consumption of the proper amounts of meat, milk and eggs will supply all the nutrients required, with or without bread.

One of the more popular misconceptions is that cheese is difficult to digest and causes constipation. This is ridiculous and libelous to a delicious, healthful and economical food.

Canned and frozen vegetables are considered to be lower in nutritive benefits than fresh vegetables. Frequently they have greater nutritive importance because vegetables can lose a considerable amount of food value during shipping and storage. On the other hand, packers take great care in canning and freezing vegetables in the freshest condition possible before they have lost appearance, flavor and nutritive value. In order to insure freshness, their processing plants are placed in proximity to the fields upon which the produce is grown.

Ours has been referred to as an age of specialists, and this applies also to the area of nutrition; universities and clinics are engaged in study and research about food values and their application to our bodies.

New and exciting information is being disseminated to

the public by means of various communications. All one has to be to benefit is receptive. Results can be noticed in the increased size of people in all enlightened countries. By increased size I am referring to height and strength, and not obesity, which unfortunately is also increasing. Longevity can, in part, be attributed to improved dietetic habits.

Foods, valuable in nutritive elements, which were once obtainable only in regions and climates in which they flourished, are now—due to improved transportation, refrigeration, and highly developed freezing processes—available to the entire nation.

The following is based on information contained in a pamphlet published by the American Dietetic Association entitled "Food Facts Talk Back."

FALLACY: Fish is "brain food."
FACT: Fish is a good wholesome food containing important nutrients for the *entire* body.

FALLACY: Coffee with cream and sugar is more harmful than black coffee.
FACT: Cream and sugar have no effect on the stimulating properties of the beverage. The only harm they do is add calories.

FALLACY: Everyone needs vitamin pills.
FACT: Everyone does *not* need vitamin pills or capsules. If a proper diet is followed, extra vitamins are superfluous, unless prescribed by a doctor for a specific reason.

FALLACY: All foods turn to fat.
FACT: Fat is formed when the total food intake exceeds the requirements of the body.

FALLACY: Banana and skim milk diet is a good method for losing weight.

FACT: This is an unhealthy diet because it is nutritionally deficient. Also, bananas are high in calories and you could consume enough to exceed your normal caloric intake.

FALLACY: The "3-day prune diet" is a good method for losing weight.

FACT: This also provides inadequate nutrition and the loss is primarily water.

FALLACY: Don't drink water while on a diet.

FACT: This is a procedure used by some "beauty farms" to obtain a quick weight loss. Any loss resulting from dehydration will soon be regained. Our bodies require water and abstinence can be dangerous.

FALLACY: Low-calorie bread should be used in all reducing diets.

FACT: Weight for weight, the caloric contents of this bread varies only slightly from regular bread.

FALLACY: Sugar is not so fattening as starch.

FACT: Weight for weight they have the same caloric value.

FALLACY: Gelatin is "non-fattening."

FACT: There is no such thing as a "fattening" or a "non-fattening" food. *All* foods contribute calories in varying amounts. Gelatin has fewer calories than, say, apple pie.

FALLACY: To reduce, eat high-protein food for a week, then the next week eat anything you want.

FACT: It is possible you would not lose *any* weight on this diet. The best procedure for weight control is a program that can be applied to a lifetime of eating—not alternate weeks.

FALLACY: Calories from meat are fattening.

FACT: Calories from one food are as fattening as an equal number from any other food. *All* protein yields 4 calories per gram.

FALLACY: Eat "Wonder Foods" such as blackstrap molasses, yogurt, brewers' yeast, wheat germ etc. to keep young and fit.

FACT: There are no "wonder foods" and those listed above are no more beneficial than many of the common foods we eat everyday. A diet containing the important nutrients is the way to better health and fitness.

FALLACY: Never give milk to a person with a fever.

FACT: Milk, as any other liquid, could help reduce the body temperature.

FALLACY: It is dangerous to leave food in an opened can.

FACT: Not true. Cover and refrigerate the food left in the can and it will preserve without damage. Foods containing acids may dissolve a little iron from the can, but this is not harmful.

FALLACY: Margarine has fewer calories than butter.

FACT: All fat yields 9 calories per gram.

FALLACY: White eggs are not so nutritious as brown eggs.

FACT: The color of the shell has no bearing on the nutritional properties of the egg.

FALLACY: Eat blackstrap molasses for anemia and rheumatism.

FACT: You couldn't possibly consume enough molasses to aid anemia. There is no evidence that any particular food will improve a rheumatic condition.

FALLACY: Home-ground flour is vastly better than com-
mercially-ground flour.

FACT: If this is to be believed then perhaps we should
obtain spinning wheels to make our own dress
fabrics.

FALLACY: Frozen orange juice is less nutritious than fresh.

FACT: They are almost identical in nutritive values.

FALLACY: Eat a grapefruit diet to reduce.

FACT: Confining yourself to one food will result in
malnutrition and leave you susceptible to
dangerous infections and disease.

9

The Bright Way to Eat

Before we discuss the specifics of the menus, please read carefully the following instructions.

DO NOT SKIP ANY MEALS OR SNACKS

You do not facilitate weight loss by eliminating any of the periodic feedings, but rather you will be disturbing the balance of the total program.

DO NOT CHANGE THE DIET BY ADDITIONS OR OMISSIONS

Each item has a particular dietetic reason for its inclusion. Any variance will cause delays in the ultimate conclusion.

DO NOT CHANGE PATTERN OF EATING SCHEDULE

The program is based on regular eating periods every 2½ or 3 hours. Do not combine meals or snacks.

Your decision to follow the program should make adherence to these instructions automatic. The eating patterns —in timing and amounts—have been clinically tested and are vital to the total concept.

Read the diet contents. Assure yourself the foods are appetizing, interesting and satisfying. The program has been proved to take off as much as 12 to 18 pounds in four to five weeks.

IMPORTANT: After reading the weekly menus, observe closely the DIRECTIONS at the end of this chapter.

WEEK 1—DAILY CONSUMPTION

Breakfast:

1 orange
    or   } alternate
½ grapefruit
1 egg—soft boiled or coddled, scrambled or fried in a teflon pan
    or
2 slices of bacon
½ piece of toast with corn oil margarine
Black coffee, tea or water. A sugar substitute may be used with coffee or tea.

Mid-Morning:

    1 cup of non-fat milk
    1 slice of American or Swiss cheese

Lunch:

    ½ can of crab
       or
    ½ can of turkey   } alternate
       or
    1 hard boiled egg
    1 serving of salad consisting of ¾ cup lettuce with
        slivers of cucumber, celery and tomato. Dressing
        consisting of 1 tablespoon of corn oil with wine
        vinegar, lemon, or any herb seasonings.
Black coffee, tea, water or diet pop

Mid-Afternoon:

    ½ cup of non-fat milk
    1 slice of American or Swiss cheese

Dinner:

1 steak, 6 oz.—broiled, dry pan fried, or
   barbequed. Worcestershire and herb
   seasonsings such as oregano, marjoram,
   basil, if desired. *No sauces or catsup*
   (this applies to all meats).
     or
1 lamb chop, 6 oz.
     or
1 pork chop, 6 oz.
     or
1 beef pattie, 6 oz.
     or
1 serving of chicken, 6 oz. broiled in foil or
   baked in foil, with wine vinegar, lemon
   or herbs

} alternate

6th and 7th day take choice of above meat
⅓ frozen package of broccoli
     or
⅓ frozen package of cauliflower
1 serving of salad consisting of ½ cup lettuce or cab-
   bage. 1 tablespoon of corn oil with wine vinegar
   or lemon and herbs
¼ can of pears
     or
¼ can of fruit cocktail
Black coffee, tea, water or diet pop

Evening:

½ cup of non-fat milk—may be mixed with hot or
   cold water—coffee, tea or diet pop
1 stalk of celery with 1 teaspoon peanut butter

WEEK 2—DAILY CONSUMPTION

Breakfast:

> 1 orange
>   or
> ½ grapefruit   } alternate
>   or
> ¼ can of peaches
> 2 strips of bacon
>   or
> 1 egg (prepare as week 1)
> ½ slice toast with corn oil margarine
> Black coffee, tea or water

Mid-Morning:

> 1 cup of non-fat milk
> 2 prunes or 1 slice of American or Swiss cheese

Lunch:

> ½ can of chicken
>   or
> ½ can of salmon   } alternate 6 days
>   or
> ½ can of shrimp
>   7th day
> 1 hard boiled egg
>
> 1 serving of salad consisting of ¾ cup of lettuce or
>   cabbage with slivers of mushroom, green peppers,
>   celery and tomato. Dressing consisting of 1 table-
>   spoon of corn oil with vinegar, or lemon and herbs.
> Black coffee, tea, water or diet pop

Mid-Afternoon:

½ cup non-fat milk
2 English walnuts, or two prunes, or 1 slice of American or Swiss cheese

Dinner:

1 serving of veal, 6 oz. (twice in the week)—broiled, dry pan fried or barbequed. Mushrooms, onion slivers, garlic, herbs, if desired. (This applies to all meats.)
 or
1 steak, 6 oz.
 or
1 lamb chop, 6 oz.
 or
1 pork chop, 6 oz. } alternate
 or
1 beef pattie, 6 oz.
 or
1 serving of chicken, 6 oz.—bake in foil, add seasonings and white wine vinegar
¼ can of string beans with 1 tablespoon of vinegar or lemon juice
 or
¼ can of sauerkraut
½ cup of salad with one tablespoon of corn oil and white wine vinegar, or lemon and herbs
¼ can of pineapple
 or
¼ can of applesauce
Black coffee, tea, water or diet pop

Evening:

   ½ cup of non-fat milk
   2 prunes

WEEK 3—DAILY CONSUMPTION

Breakfast:

   1 orange   ⎤
        or   ⎬ alternate
   ¼ can of apricots ⎦
   1 egg (prepare as week 1)
        or
   2 sausages
   ½ slice of bread with corn oil margarine
   Black coffee, tea or water

Mid-Morning:

   1 cup of non-fat milk
   1 slice of American or Swiss cheese

Lunch:

   ½ of a 5¾ oz. can of turkey ⎤
        or   ⎥
   ½ can of tuna   ⎬ alternate
        or   ⎥
   ½ can of crab   ⎦
   1 tomato with 1 tablespoon of corn oil
        or
   ¾ cup of shredded lettuce with 1 tablespoon of corn
        oil, vinegar or lemon and herbs
   Black coffee, tea, water or diet pop

Mid-Afternoon:

½ cup of non-fat milk
2 prunes or 2 English walnuts

Dinner:

1 serving steak, 6 oz.—broiled, dry pan
fried or barbequed. Herb seasonings
and Worcestershire, if desired. (This
applies to all meats.)
  or
1 lamb chop, 6 oz.
  or
1 pork chop, 6 oz.
  or
1 serving of veal, 6 oz.
  or
1 beef pattie, 6 oz.

} alternate

1 serving of white fish, 6 oz. (Two days in week—
on days fish not served at lunch.)
¼ can of spinach
  or
¼ can of asparagus
½ cup of salad with 1 tablespoon corn oil with wine
vinegar, or lemon and herbs
¼ can of pears
  or
¼ can of grapefruit
Black coffee, tea, water or diet pop

Evening:

½ cup of non-fat milk
1 celery stalk with 1 teaspoon peanut butter

WEEK 4—DAILY CONSUMPTION

Breakfast:

>   1 orange
>   1 breakfast steak, 4 oz. broiled or dry pan fried
>   or
>   1 egg (prepare as week 1)
>   ½ slice of bread with corn oil margarine
>   Black coffee, tea or water

Mid-Morning:

>   2 prunes
>   1 cup of non-fat milk

Lunch:

>   ½ of 5¾ oz. can of boned chicken ⎫
>   or   ⎪
>   ½ can of salmon   ⎬ alternate
>   or   ⎪
>   ½ can of shrimp   ⎭
>   ¾ cup of lettuce or cabbage salad, with slivers of to-
>   mato, green pepper and celery. Add 1 tablespoon
>   of corn oil with vinegar or lemon and herbs
>   Black coffee, tea, water or diet pop

Mid-Afternoon:

>   ½ cup of non-fat milk
>   1 slice of American or Swiss cheese

Dinner:

1 lamb chop, 6 oz. broiled, dry pan fried or
    barbequed. Marinate in wine vinegar
    and herbs, if desired. (This applies to
    all meats.)
    or
1 pork chop, 6 oz.
    or
1 serving of veal, 6 oz.   alternate
    or
1 serving of chicken, 6 oz. bake in foil, add
    seasonings and white wine vinegar
    or
1 beef pattie, 6 oz.
    or
1 serving of white fish, 6 oz.—bake in foil add sea-
    sonings and white wine vinegar. (Two times in
    week when not eaten at lunch.)
¼ can of string beans
    or
¼ can of tomatoes
½ cup of green salad with 1 tablespoon of corn oil with
    wine vinegar or lemon and herbs
¼ can of apricots
    or
¼ can of applesauce
Black coffee, tea, water or diet pop

Evening:

½ cup of non-fat milk
1 slice of American or Swiss cheese

DIRECTIONS

Cheese servings should be 1" x 2½" x ⅛".

Margarine quantity for morning toast should be ½ pat.

Follow *all* quantities as specified. Increasing the amounts will retard or prevent weight loss. If you eat more than the allowed portion of meat one night, reduce the portion the following night.

All fruits must be either fresh or low-calorie canned.

If desired, sprinkle ¼ teaspoon of grated Parmesan cheese on the salads.

Although this is not a salt-free diet, it is not advisable to add salt or monosodium glutamate. If salt is needed, use it sparingly.

Several methods are suggested for preparing the meat to offer variety and flavor. If one is preferred over the others, it is permissible to use it for all servings.

You may use onion or garlic powder (not salt), if desired on meats and vegetables.

Continue following the four weeks program until you have reached your desired weight.

10

Off . . . For Keeps

If this program didn't offer a means for maintaining the loss, it would lack a fundamental purpose for its existence. Earlier in the book I mentioned that, on again—off again on again diet attempts could be more harmful than a sustained state of moderate overweight. If the precepts of the program are observed you will leave it off . . . for keeps.

Once you have reduced to your preferred weight the period of greatest discipline is behind you. The maintenance program allows considerable latitude. This does not mean you can be indiscriminate, but you can be relaxed.

By the time you have concluded the reducing part of the program you will have become familiar enough with the concept of the diet to understand what we are trying to do nutritionally. You won't have to continue to follow prescribed menus, or count quantities, or even measure portions. You will *know*, without being reminded, when you are overindulging. If there is any doubt, your scales or your tape measure will affirm or deny.

It should not be necessary to remind people having suffered the discomforts of obesity that they have a propensity for accumulating fat. Most people have to watch their weight to some degree, but those having experienced 20 or more pounds of excess weight must be ever vigilant.

Continue to weigh and measure yourself regularly, as a small increase can be easily corrected. Proceed cautiously in expanding your intake. The next few weeks will be of great importance. If you should "shock" your metabolism with a sudden large dose of carbohydrates you could suffer a major gain.

The following is presented to you as a guide for a gradual increase back to a normal diet. They can be added to any of the weekly menus outlined in Chapter 9.

MAINTENANCE PROGRAM
(following weight reduction)

WEEK 1 ADD

1. ½ slice of bread to breakfast + ½ pat of margarine. (Making a total of 1 slice with 1 pat.)
2. Another vegetable to your dinner.

If there is no gain in weight, keep the above in your diet and,

WEEK 2 ADD

1. A fruit for lunch.
2. Potato for dinner, or if preferred, rice or macaroni.

If there is no gain in weight, keep all the above in your diet and,

WEEK 3 ADD

1. *Once* this week, eat something you desire more than anything else. Perhaps one of those tidbits you have been denying yourself.

2. Increase slightly the quantity of meats and vegetables.

NOTE: In Appendix III you will find two lists of vegetables. List I should take preference in your maintenance program. There is also a list of common foods comparable in caloric value to one slice of bread.

If, after the above additions to your diet, you show no gain in either weight or measurements, you can be confident you have achieved the desired adjustment in your metabolism.

You should now be able to eat just about everything—in moderate amounts. Hopefully you will no longer crave the "gooey" things you ate in the past. Your new knowledge should help you choose the right foods in the right amounts.

Most people will lose their compulsion to overeat—being on a perfectly balanced program (often for the first time) they no longer have the desire for gluttony.

Let me explain the purpose for continuing the periodic feedings—three meals, three snacks. Its primary function is to avoid a severe drop in energy level. The stomach empties itself every four hours. To anticipate this and to preclude a sudden drop in blood sugar level (energy) I suggest you continue to eat in two and a half to three hour intervals.

Most of you have experienced that mid-morning, or mid-afternoon "letdown." This results from your blood sugar dropping below full energy level. The "letdown" *is* a physical condition.

This program does not require you to concern yourself

with counting calories. (Calories *do* count but I do the counting for you). Continue eating the types of foods recommended in the program. This will not only maintain your weight but also keep you well-nourished.

NOTE: One of the questions asked frequently by people contemplating beginning the program is: "Am I allowed to drink?" The answer is *yes*.

It will not affect your progress on the diet to have a drink or two before dinner, if you confine the drinking to bourbon, scotch, gin or vodka and *water*. Or, you may have the above beverages "on the rocks." Do not drink cocktails such as manhattans, daiquiris, etc. A lemon or lime twist may be added, if desired. Do not drink beer or wine.

11

Top to Toe Tone-Up

Exercising will not make the overweight slender. Reducing by strenuous bodily exertion is virtually impossible as well as highly impractical. A young athlete may remain slender while actively engaged in sports, but this is due as much to his well adjusted metabolism as from his energetic pursuits. "In training" consists of a highly nutritious diet with a minimum of sweets and pastries.

Occasionally, however, even young athletes are placed on diets. During training seasons this means being relegated to the "fat man's table." In spite of their vigorous physical program, they cannot eat indiscriminately and still maintain most efficient weight. Thus we can dispel any theory relating to exercise rather than diet for reducing.

However, moderate exercise is essential in a body improvement program. It is important for stimulating circulation and firming muscle tissues.

The exercises I am recommending are not strenuous and

take only minutes a day. They are applicable to men and women, the weak and the strong, because the exertion expended is in proportion to a person's strength and physical make-up. They are based, primarily, on isometrics, which means you are exerting against your own strength and resistance. A 200 pound man will exert proportionately more power, or pressure, than a 120 pound woman.

It is important to do them *every* day. You will not gain the benefits by attempting to double or triple them every two or three days, or make up for the week on Saturday. They are designed for regularity and it is far easier to form the habit if you do them each day at the same time of the day. You will find them enjoyable rather than tedious or difficult—stimulating rather than tiring.

The number of times recommended for each exercise is the minimum; as your body gets accustomed to the routine they should be increased.

Even at the most leisurely pace they should not involve more than ten minutes of your day. Results will convince you your time was never better spent.

FOREHEAD

Place each forefinger on outer edge of each eyebrow, exert pressure toward ears—now try to frown. Repeat 5 times.

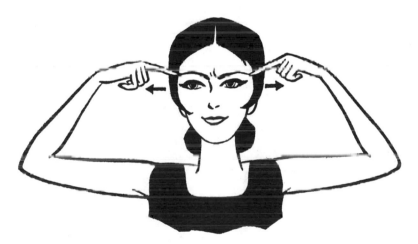

EYES—CROW'S-FEET

Place forefingers on outer corner of each eye—exert upward pressure while trying to look down. Repeat 7 times.

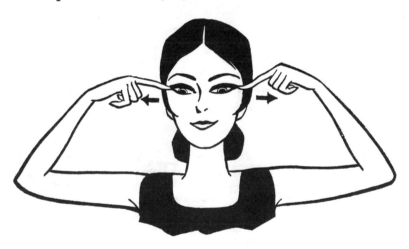

MOUTH AND LOWER FACE

Say "Wahoo"—opening and closing mouth as far as possible each time. Repeat 7 times.

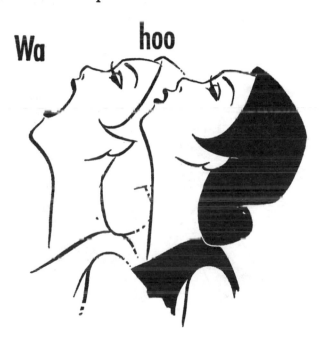

NECK AND JAWLINE

Throw head back as far as possible. Make "pop" sound. Repeat 5 times. With your head thrown back, turn to left and repeat 5 times. Next to the right and repeat 5 times. Turn head only and not the body.

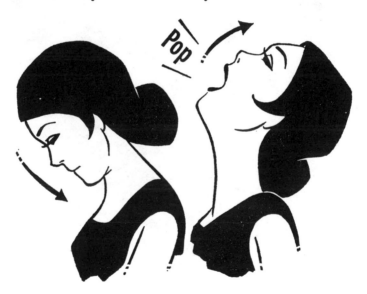

UPPER ARM

Stretch arms above head as far as possible. "Dry swim" pulling vigorously each arm alternately. Repeat 5 times with each arm.

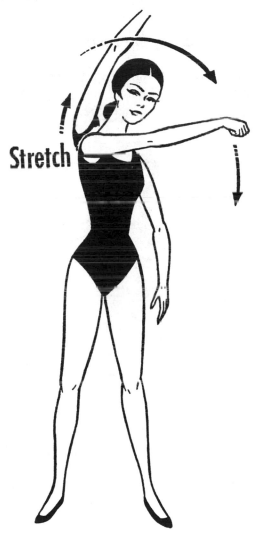

CHEST AND BUSTLINE

Raise elbows to chest level. Press finger tips together as hard as possible, until you feel the pull in pectoral and abdominal muscles. Release and repeat 7 times.

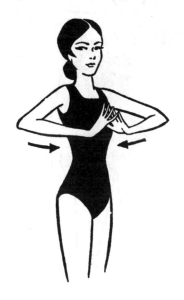

WAIST

Left arm straight up over your head. Right arm straight
down by your side. Stretch bend to the right as far as possible. Return erect and repeat 5 times. Now reverse the arm
position and repeat 5 times to the left.

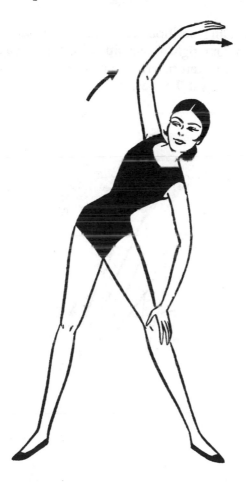

BACK

From a standing position, cross your feet and with knees
stiff, stretch your right finger tips as far as possible toward
your right toes. Return erect and repeat 7 times. Now the
left side and repeat 7 times.

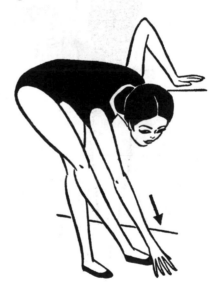

STOMACH

Place hands on hips. "Pull in" your stomach as far as possible. Release pressure. Repeat 7 times.

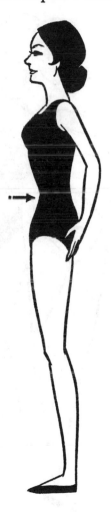

HIPS

Stand perpendicular to a hard, flat wall. Arms straight out in front of you. "Knock on wall" with your left hip 7 times. Repeat on right side.

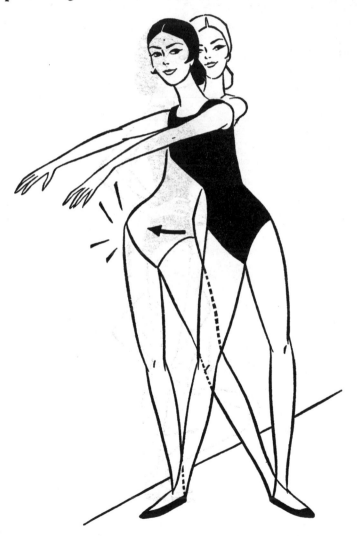

THIGHS

Place hands on hips. Do 7 deep knee bends, returning to standing position each time. Use only thigh muscles to return.

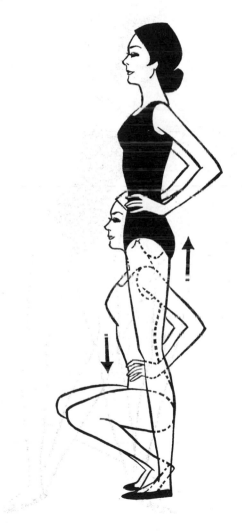

CALF, ANKLE, FEET

Stand straight with your feet flat on the floor, about 8 inches apart. Now turn toes inward. Raise up on toes and down again, repeating 10 times.

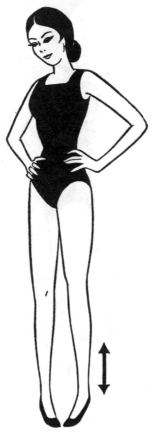

12

What's Your Girth Worth?

Those undesirable pounds are the most costly part of your body.

I am not referring to the cost of the food it took to put you in the shape you're in. I am referring to the price you pay in loss of energy; the detriment to your appearance; the hazards to your health. I am referring to the anxiety and discomfort you experience; the embarrassing stares you invite; the price of lost pride and self-confidence.

The slender are the envied—the fat are the pitied.

Only five per cent of you have a medical reason for being fat; the rest of you can do something about it.

Is self-indulgence worth the price you pay in loss of dignity? Let me assure you it is a rare fat man or woman who looks dignified.

Is your girth worth the huffing and puffing, not of walking up stairs, but just walking? Is it worth the image you view in your mirror, or the discomforting tightness of your belt, or the bulges no well-fitted dress can hide?

There is indisputable medical evidence that your girth may be worth years of your life.

There is also considerable evidence that your girth may be depriving you of enjoyment in the years you do live.

People not cursed with overweight are not necessarily blessed with a naturally slender physique. Oh, I know there are people whose weight doesn't seem to vary in spite of constant gourmandizing, but these are as rare as those whose overweight is due to physiological reasons. A sensible eating pattern preserves most figures. The majority have to make a constant effort to keep their weight down. You will note people adjusting their intake for a day or two after there has been unusually heavy eating as a holiday or a special evening out.

Many people put weight on during a vacation, but will make a determined effort to watch their intake the following weeks. I have heard slender people remark they take off pounds prior to the Christmas holidays, or Passover, in anticipation of the bounties available during these days of feasting.

You may not think the anticipation of a life of privation worth the effort, but be assured it is worth every sacrifice you may *think* you are making. A weight maintenance program need not be a grim endeavor. If you can control your indulgences and compensate for it during succeeding days, you can occasionally eat those delights that are forbidden during the actual weight reducing period. By the time you have lost your excessive layers of fat and your metabolism has adjusted to normality you will become your own best guardian of the flesh.

Is your girth worth the guilt that accompanies a visit to your doctor? Although his concern is only for your health, many people will resent his intrusion into their private arena of fat. Guilt promotes this resentment.

How often I have heard people remark that their resistance to a medical check-up results from knowing exactly what he is going to say—"You're too heavy." We will quickly take his advice and his prescriptions if it relates to something organic such as our kidneys or our headaches or our "sour" stomach. All of our ailments may relate directly or indirectly to obesity, but yet we resent references to it.

I am acquainted with a man who sensibly has a thorough checkup each year. He has a marked tendency toward obesity, but each year, a few weeks prior to his appointment, he will put himself on a starvation diet to avoid chastisement by his doctor. To tell him this is childish and unhealthy would only be inviting his wrath.

Paraphrasing a biblical quotation, a doctor has a sign hanging in his office which reads, "What does it profiteth a man if he gains, and loses his health?"

13

Helps, Hints, Hopes

Your determined effort to reduce may need encouragement and occasional stimulation. It will help to read Chapter 15 where you might find examples closely paralleling your own circumstance. To know there are many who have reached a happy conclusion should make you realize this reward is also within your reach.

Following the program conscientiously for even two weeks will demonstrate sufficient results to compensate for any sacrifice you feel you might be enduring. Almost invariably there is testimony to "feeling better" even before there is a noticeable weight loss. This, of course, results from being better nourished. Dramatic changes in dimensions and weight begin to occur in three to four weeks. Experience has evinced overwhelming evidence to prove those following the program for this length of time will seldom regress unless there are psychological influences to upset their good intentions.

It is necessary to avoid experiences that might be traumatic. Domestic conflicts can trigger a setback. These situations cannot always be avoided, and certainly you can't ignore an uncomfortable plight merely by my suggesting you do so. I can only tell you to develop your resolve to the point where you will not *allow* anything to deter you.

You have set a goal of your own volition and only your efforts can bring about attainment. If you are tempted to succumb to an eating spree for any reason, try resisting by positive thoughts involving the benefits you have already enjoyed in the time you have been reducing. Be selfish or egotistical about it. Think only of the pleasant benefits accruing to you. Look at other fat people and take pride in what you are achieving. Consider all the disadvantages of being overweight and the advantages of being slender. Consider the additional time and effort a setback will entail.

The word "diet" invokes an unattractive image. As I stated in the beginning of this book, most of you, having interest enough to read and embrace this program, have ventured into many methods and thus consider the word "diet" an anathema.

Perhaps if we used the Greek derivation of the word, *diaita*, meaning, "manner of living," it would become more palatable to you. I hope by reading this book and understanding the processes of the program you will realize that I am literally discussing a manner of living and not merely the dissolving of unwanted pounds.

Good health, a feeling of well-being, the energy for enjoying varied pleasant interests are certainly bountiful contributions toward a "manner of living." Or perhaps I should say a *new* manner of living.

The program is relatively simple and provides ample amounts of food for both men and women. To aid you in making it as convenient as possible I suggest you prepare, in advance, each week's portions in daily amounts. This will even include slicing bread in the recommended portion. Place those foods requiring freezing in the freezer and defrost daily rations each morning.

By following this procedure, you not only make it easy to prepare each meal and snack, but it has proved to be a great help in keeping within the recommended amounts. I have noticed quantities may vary when each meal or snack is prepared individually.

If the dieter is a working man or woman, place the required amount of non-fat milk powder in a piece of wax paper and carry with other snack items. It will be simple to dilute the milk in a paper cup at the water fountain.

The importance of preparing food portions in advance has led me to supply my patients with the necessary items as they visit each week at my office. It relieves them of one more detail, and I have found it helps greatly for them to be as free as possible from unnecessary details. This is particularly important during the initial weeks of the program when new eating habits are being formed.

Plan your own procedures to make it as easy as possible for *you*. You are offered a selection of meat for the evening meal. Try to eat the variety but if you do not like pork chops then substitute one of the other choices. However, it is important that you do not eliminate the fish, poultry and veal from the diet. Herbs are recommended because they can sometimes make the difference between "another" piece of meat and a gourmet delicacy.

It is inevitable that some people will have periods of regression. If this happens to you it is important you feel no remorse. Most obese people have a guilt complex about eating. If you get an urge to deviate from the diet, try talking yourself out of it, or thinking yourself out of it; but if the urge is irresistible it is better to have a momentary relapse than discontinuing the program altogether. Just realize you will lose some ground and prepare yourself for it to avoid discouragement.

Here is a procedure I find is frequently successful in overcoming temptation—take whatever goodie is craved and face a mirror. Look at yourself as you take a bite or a spoonful. It is very likely this will discourage you from eating it.

A major benefit of this program, and an important difference from the highly publicized diets, is permanent weight loss. This results in the change which takes place in your metabolism. This change occurs from two important elements in the program—the choice of food *and* the pattern of eating. The latter is equally as important as the food and that is why this is a weight reducing "program"—not merely a "diet." To keep your weight at the desired level, you must continue to observe the eating schedule, including the snacks.

Although you will not be able to go back to your old eating habits, and indeed you will not want to, your body will be able to assimilate a moderate amount of high caloric food without developing fat at its previous rate.

14

Tomorrow and Tomorrow
and Tomorrow

The mores of our society demand discipline in every facet of our lives, from answering the morning alarm to brewing the morning coffee to putting the cat out at night.

Living in our society does not permit lapses in self-control. Many of these impositions are so habitual that we are not necessarily aware of them as disciplines. Mother knows she has to have dinner ready at 6:00; she knows the weekly wash has to be done. Father doesn't question having to be in the office five days a week. These are patterns of normal living and do not necessarily associate themselves with the obvious discipline of maintaining a weight watching program.

Don't handicap yourself by needless self-pity. Think of a careful nutritional pattern as another necessity for abundant living. And indeed it is. Your shame, your guilt, and your lassitude will disappear with the layers of fat; and as the fat melts away, your enthusiasm for life and its activities will replace and compensate for any imagined joy you received from your former eating orgies and self-indulgence.

Don't feel martyred. You are not giving anything up. You are making an important adjustment to a fuller, more meaningful life with all the happiness that accompanies a prideful, attractive body. All you have left behind are mountains of ugly, unnecessary fat. Your reward is greater comfort and a healthier physique.

Don't let discouragement set you back in your resolve. Don't let emotional problems lead you again to overeating. Gourmandizing didn't help before so don't be mislead into thinking it might again. A healthy vigorous body is far better equipped, physically and emotionally, to deal with problems.

This is a book on self-improvement and is therefore meant to be used as a constant reminder and stimulant. Don't lose it on a bookshelf or in a drawer; keep it where you can see it and reach for it for daily guidance and help. Keep your chart handy and continue to weigh and measure yourself regularly. Pounds can sneak up on us stealthily and insidiously. Be constantly vigilant. Checking a gain of several pounds can be painless and quick. The sudden realization of a 20-pound increase can be ruinous.

Remind yourself that you are not a minority of one that has to watch his diet but rather belong to the vast majority of 85 per cent who require a handy scale to keep an attractive figure.

When you have reached your proper weight you have achieved one of the most important goals in your life— because it may well mean life for you.

Congratulations and happy health tomorrow and tomorrow and tomorrow.

15

The Winning Losers

Those who have sought my help fall into no specific social, ethnic or economic classification. There is no pattern of occupation or age. Patients have ranged from the young to the elderly; from extreme cases of obesity to those desiring changes in measurements with little weight loss.

Male patients have included doctors, stockbrokers, filling station attendants, businessmen and salesmen.

They include the affluent and those confined to a taut budget. There are those with diabetes and respiratory ailments. I am not a physician; I am a dietitian, and thus any claims made concerning patients receiving relief from physical disorders are normal reactions resulting from the loss of weight and a proper diet. Numerous are the physical problems resulting from poor eating habits and overweight.

I have people who have been pressured by their families and others who have started the program without the knowledge of their husband or wife. Patients have been referred to me by internists, psychologists, psychiatrists, marriage counselors and clergymen.

However, the most gratifying referrals are from those who have experienced the rewards of the program.

There is no more convincing authentication of a program of self-improvement than the actual evidence of successful conclusions and results. A feeling of inadequacy comes over me as I try to put into words the delight and enthusiasm of those who have realized their goal. How do you express the sparkle in their eyes, the glow on their face, the exuberance of newly found energy.

Satisfaction from accomplishment is self-rewarding. To know you have conquered an obstacle, particularly one that has been plaguing you for years, is a satisfying experience. To have demonstrated will-power and achieved an emotional, psychological and physiological victory is indeed a gratifying sensation.

The case histories do not necessarily include the extreme cases, but rather a cross section of ages, weights and psychological influences.

Because the tape measure is as important as the scales, measurements are included in most cases.

Let the following examples be an inspiration.

The young wife of an internist came to me with a familiar pessimistic attitude. "I was born fat, grew up fat, and am convinced I will always be fat."

She is 5'1" and on October 3 weighed 159½ pounds. By the first of January she was down to 127½ pounds with remarkable adjustments in her measurements. On the day she reached 127½ she came in with one of her cute, mischievous grins and said, "I've decided to be mad at you. My mother gave me a beautiful dress last fall and I have been saving it for a special occasion. The occasion came last Saturday, and when I tried it on it hung on me like a muu-muu."

Before		After
12	Arms	10½
38	Bust	34
33½	Rib cage	28½
34	Waist	27½
42	Stomach	34
44	Hips	34
23½	Thighs	20¾

A woman approached me after a lecture I delivered at a women's club. She lamented having tried "diet after diet after diet" during the past ten years. She had exhausted her patience and endurance and was prepared to accept her fate. However, my program sounded so sensible to her she decided "to give it one more go."

She reduced from 167 pounds to 129½, and her face was radiant as she said, "I know I will never be heavy again." She is within 5 pounds of her desired weight and though she now "cheats" occasionally, she continues to make progress.

In less than four months the following changes in her measurements took place:

Before		After
13	Arms	10⅝
40	Bust	37
35	Rib cage	30
34	Waist	28
38¾	Stomach	35
43	Hips	37
25	Thighs	21¼
15	Calf	13½
9¾	Ankle	8¾

A thirty-seven year old wife of a business executive weighed 177½ pounds, and after years of obesity decided to do something about it. Increasing periods of depression resulted from feeling ill at ease and conspicuous in social gatherings. Her husband's business involved entertainment and social obligations in which wives participated. She became less and less "available" for these events.

The climax to her problem and the deep hurt to her pride that led her to my clinic occurred when she overheard a woman acquaintance refer to her as "dowdy." She had always taken great pride in her grooming and clothes, but excessive weight discouraged her from continued faithfulness to personal care. Now she was finally motivated to take action.

By May 18, just three months after beginning the program she was down to 139 pounds and subsequently reduced to 130½, the weight she is maintaining.

Her social life has resumed and she entertained a large group for a surprise birthday party for her husband. Included among the guests was the acquaintance she heard call her "dowdy." She now considers her a friend.

Before		After
14	Arms	12
39½	Bust	35¼
35	Waist	27½
42½	Stomach	34
44	Hips	37¼
26	Thighs	21

The age of a person has no effect on the results. A man of sixty-six who had recently retired brought his weight down from 217 pounds to 185 in three months with the following important changes in measurements:

Before		After
15¾	Neck	15
13	Arms	12½
42	Chest	40
40½	Waist	36½
41½	Hips	40

He has had little trouble maintaining his weight despite much traveling.

Another man who reduced from 209 pounds to 180 in two months reduced his waist from 42 inches to 36 inches. At the same time his neck measurement went from 17½ inches to 15½ inches.

It might appear that it is a great deal easier to lose weight if you prepare all the meals yourself. This is generally true; however, one woman who went from 163½ pounds to 138½ pounds in nine weeks *ate out every night*.

I remember, with particular pleasure, a forty-three year old grandmother who checked in at 5'2" and 122½ pounds. Hers was not so much a weight problem as a figure problem, with noticeable fat deposits around the rib cage, waist, hips and thighs. Her total weight loss was only 8½ pounds, but look what happened to her measurements, in only two months.

Before		After
10½	Arms	10½
34	Bust	34
32	Rib cage	29
26⅞	Waist	24¼
32⅜	Stomach	31¼
36¾	Hips	34
22¾	Thighs	19
12¾	Calf	12½
7½	Ankle	7½

It is generally accepted that the ideal female measurements is for the waist to be 10 inches less than the bust and the hips the same size as the bust. Although this woman lost only 8½ pounds she lost them where they had accumulated to achieve a figure that is even better proportioned "than when I was a teenager."

Another remarkable change in dimensions with little weight loss involved a woman fifty-nine years of age, 5 feet and weighing only 111 pounds. The weight loss was negligible but the effect the program had on her measurements was dramatic. This took place between May 26 and July 15.

Before		After
37¼	Bust	35¼
30⅛	Rib cage	27¾
28⅛	Waist	26
35½	Hips	34½
17⅞	Thighs	17½

A young woman of twenty-nine was directed to me by her physician. She was 5'7" and at 280½ pounds suffered from dangerously high blood pressure. Her blood pressure and lassitude resulting from severe obesity made her unable to work. In twelve weeks her weight had dropped 41½ pounds.

Although she has experienced two setbacks her weight has reached 201. The progress has been so encouraging there should be little doubt that she will eventually reduce to an acceptable weight.

Her blood pressure, although not yet normal, is no longer at the danger point. She is now employed and for the first time in many years is involved in a social life.

Before		After
Before		*After*
19	Arms	13½
53	Bust	38½
45½	Waist	37
56	Hips	43
30½	Thighs	21½
19¼	Calf	15¼

It is medically accepted that there is a correlation between diabetes and obesity. In one particular case this was proved dramatically. A thirty-eight year old diabetic, weighing 159 pounds, was referred to me by her doctor.

She reduced to 118 pounds, and, on advice of her physician, discontinued her insulin medication.

A woman suffering from uncontrolled diabetes at the age of fifty-six and 176½ pounds, started the program, on the advice of her doctor on June 14. By August 28 she was down to 145½ pounds and her diabetes was in control. She was placed, by her physician, on smaller amounts of insulin to be taken orally rather than by injection.

A short while ago a patient was referred to me who had been going to a "diet" doctor daily for "shots." In addition she was taking numerous pills prescribed by this same doctor. One day she told the nurse she would be unable to report in for her shot the next day. To compensate for this she was given a "double shot." When she got home her throat swelled (laryngeal edema) and she almost choked to death. A doctor from the building in which I have my clinic was called. He was able to save her life, and advised her to use my program. She is now achieving a satisfactory weight loss without medication.

I was very interested in an experience I had with a mother and daughter. They came in together. The mother weighed 165 and her fourteen year old daughter, 158. The mother explained, "I finally am determined to take off weight, and induced Dorothy to join me. I thought we would have a better chance for success if we undertook it together."

This is an excellent plan and I have seen it work successfully with fathers and sons as well as mothers and daughters. In this case, however, both of them did not finish the program. The mother, who "induced Dorothy to join me" dropped out after six weeks while the daughter continued until she lost 30 pounds and the following inches:

Bust	3 inches
Rib cage	2 inches
Waist	5 inches
Hips	4¾ inches
Thighs	4½ inches

Until the program is completed and you are adjusted to the maintenance program, disappointing setbacks can occur. One man who had taken off 22 pounds in six weeks went on a two week vacation and put back 13 pounds.

A woman weighing in at 245 pounds lost 25 pounds in five weeks. She suffered a traumatic shock in the loss of a pet dog and it took her five months to remove another 25 pounds.

Here is another example of dramatic change in measurements. This woman started at 175 and by the time she reached 140 she had removed the following inches:

	Loss in inches
Neck	1¼
Arm	2
Bust	3
Rib cage	4½

Waist	4½
Stomach	5½
Hips	5½
Buttocks	7
Thigh	5½
Knee	4
Calf	2
Ankle	½

Don't you think it is worth small sacrifices for results like these? Those who have experienced the rewards are evangelistic in their praise of the program.

A woman who weighed only 114, was troubled with bulges on her rib cage, waist and hips. By removing only six pounds the following changes occurred:

Before		*After*
30½	Rib cage	26½
27½	Waist	25¾
36	Hips	34

This is further evidence that the program's importance is not only weight loss but inches lost.

You *too* can "Eat Yourself Slim."

Appendix I

DESIRABLE WEIGHTS FOR WOMEN 25 AND OVER*
(Weight According to Frame—In Indoor Clothing)

HEIGHT† feet inches	SMALL FRAME	MEDIUM FRAME	LARGE FRAME
4 10	92–98	96–107	104–119
4 11	94–101	98–110	106–122
5 0	96–104	101–113	109–125
5 1	99–107	104–116	112–128
5 2	102–110	107–119	115–131
5 3	105–113	110–122	118–134
5 4	108–116	113–126	121–138
5 5	111–119	116–130	125–142
5 6	114–123	120–135	129–146
5 7	118–127	124–139	133–150
5 8	122–131	128–143	137–154
5 9	126–135	132–147	141–158
5 10	130–140	136–151	145–163
5 11	134–144	140–155	149–168
6 0	138–148	144–159	153–173

† with shoes on—2-inch heels

DESIRABLE WEIGHTS FOR MEN 25 AND OVER*
(Weight According to Frame—In Indoor Clothing)

HEIGHT‡ feet inches	SMALL FRAME	MEDIUM FRAME	LARGE FRAME
5 2	112–120	118–129	126–141
5 3	115–123	121–133	129–144
5 4	118–126	124–136	132–148
5 5	121–129	127–139	135–152
5 6	124–133	130–143	138–156
5 7	128–137	134–147	142–161
5 8	132–141	138–152	147–166
5 9	136–145	142–156	151–170
5 10	140–150	146–160	155–174
5 11	144–154	150–165	159–179
6 0	148–158	154–170	164–184
6 1	152–162	158–175	168–189
6 2	156–167	162–180	173–194
6 3	160–171	167–185	178–199
6 4	164–175	172–190	182–204

‡ with shoes on—1-inch heels
* Data prepared by Metropolitan Life Insurance Company.

Appendix II

Measurement chart

Week	Start	1	2	3	4	5	6	7	8
Weight									
Arms									
Bust									
Rib cage									
Waist									
Stomach									
Hips									
Thighs									
Calves									
Ankle									

Appendix III

VEGETABLE LIST I

Low in carbohydrates, protein and calories

Asparagus	Mushrooms
Broccoli	Radishes
Cabbage	Sauerkraut
Cauliflower	Spinach
Celery	Summer Squash
Cucumbers	Tomatoes
Lettuce	Watercress

VEGETABLE LIST II

Higher in carbohydrates, protein and calories

Artichokes	Onions
Beets	Peppers
Carrots	Pumpkin
Green beans	Rutabagas
Wax beans	Turnips
Green peas	Winter Squash

Each of the following, in specified amounts, are equivalent in carbohydrates, protein and calories.

Bread	1 slice
Cereal, cooked	½ cup
Cereal, dry	¾ cup
Rice, grits, cooked	½ cup
Spaghetti, noodles, cooked	½ cup
Crackers, graham	2
Crackers, saltines	5
Potatoes, white	1 small
Potatoes, white, mashed	½ cup
Potatoes, sweet or Yam	¼ cup
Beans or peas, dried or cooked	½ cup
Baked beans without pork	¼ cup
Corn	⅓ cup

Index